I0449617

The IROKO Tree

African roots meet ancient India
for wellbeing

Ligia Braz, Rondy Isaac

& Sandra de Moura

Ligia Braz, Rondy Isaac & Sandra de Moura

The IROKO Tree

African roots meet ancient India
for wellbeing

First Edition
Stuttgart, Palo Alto, Tuscaloosa 2017
ISBN 978-1-326-90613-9

The IROKO Tree

African roots meet ancient India

for wellbeing

Ligia Braz, Rondy Isaac

& Sandra de Moura

Publisher: Brasiversum & lulu.com

© 2017. Stuttgart, Germany

Graphics & Cover: Ligia Braz

Pictures: Sandra de Moura, Rondy Isaac

Printed by Lulu.com

ISBN 978-1-326-90613-9

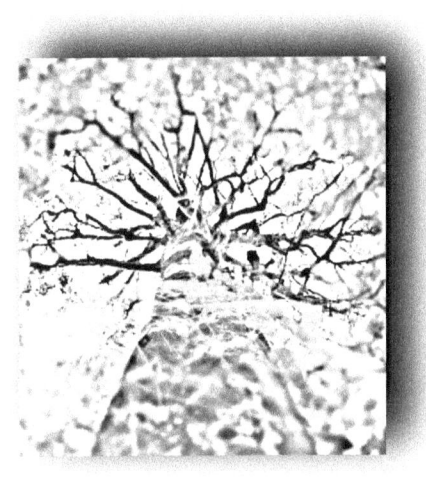

We dedicate this work

to all the ancestors,

especially the ones

originating in Africa.

Thankfulness for:

- *all our teachers during our life, for inspiring us to seek and find our true selfs*

- *the brotherhood and love between us that we would like to share with you*

- *all relatives and friends that have supported us*

- *for you opening, reading, and using this book*

Introduction

The illusion of time.

The intuition of the way.
The now and the eternity.
The whole and the individual.

In search of the roots, understanding, and a healthy basis for life. We came across the Iroko tree. At this moment, we found much more than another metaphor, we found the roots and the comprehension of our own ways, a history with a beginning, content and end, guiding the compilation of ancient knowledge and lessons acquired during a lifetime. It is like a foundation for well being!

Who are we:

Sandra de Moura, Brazilian, born in Recife, German, resident of Tuscaloosa, Alabama, Personal Trainer, Yoga teacher.

Rondy Isaac, American, born in Los Angeles, resides in the San Francisco bay area, Holistic Nutritionist, Yoga Teacher.

Ligia Braz, Brazilian, born in São Paulo, German, resident of Esslingen, social worker, writer, journalist, life coach specialist in integrative hypnosis based in neuroscience.

Our goals:

Beyond the search for inner peace for the time we live in, a constant bombardment of information and stimulations, we seek wellness through easy, pleasant, and quick exercises to be performed regularly.

We wish for ourselves and everyone that wants to come along, to find relief from stress, pain, anxiety, fear, and insecurity that can appear, at any moment, in the lives of each one of us.

What we propose:

A daily thought of self-compassion, some minutes to be dedicated for yourself, exploring your body, your mind, and spiritual world.

In this booklet, we demonstrate some possibilities of these exercises, plunging into the inspiring Afro-America cultures, that we all 3 of us have in common.

What we want:

May you be happy!
May your path be steady and smooth.
May love flow

... and may self-compassion take root, grow, develop, and flourish for all human beings.

The Iroko Tree

The Iroko Tree

No other country in our world synthesizes African culture like Brazil.

Africa is a huge continent, full of different cultures, languages and traditions.

In Brazil, African cultures are integrated throughout society. In the United States and the Americas (north, south and central) African culture is prominent.

The heritage of African mythology continues to live in the Americas, the summary of the culture of that continent, where all humanity are said to come from.

The Iroko tree can be found today in West Africa. It is an strong and very tall tree with many branches, like the African culture. Its wood is used in the manufacture of furniture and also for building houses. It has a important mythology of its own. Even though this mythology was carried across the Atlantic, many of us lost the connection to our roots. The Iroko tree was the conduit for the Orisha's descending to earth. Orisha, is African word for Spirit God. They are still worshipped today in many countries of the America's.

Metaphors with trees symbolizing life, protection, strength and peace can be found in many religions. Even in some lifestyles, more linked to nature, trees play a key role in the human imagination.

This tree, for the oldest African civilizations, meant the bridge between heaven and earth. Between our world and the world of spirits and gods. It is through the tree of Iroko that all the other gods, many of them known in Brazil and in other parts of the world, as the Orishas of candomblé or umbanda. It is through strong roots grounded firmly in the earth and many high branches touching the sky, that the inspiration, the answers, the archetypes, the symbols, and the metaphors, become conscious and real. The process is clear. The metaphor heaven and earth, conscious and unconscious, human and divine, among many others, become our paved road for well being.

Details of the Tree

In Africa they believe, the tree known as "Iroko", is the first tree to be planted on Earth.
It is known as *Milicia Excelsa*. It can reach 45 meters in height and 3m in diameter.
In Brazil, the Iroko tree does not exist, but the tree of Iroko is known as *Ficus Gomelleira*. Or commonly known as *Gameleira*, a tree of strong, multiple roots, that is frequently found near the riverbanks. Its is impressive although its not as tall as the Iroko tree.

Details on the Iroko deity

Iroko is a divinity that represents ancestry, while it is also the home of all other deities. He is the master of time and space. To disrespect Iroko means to disrespect our own origins, our family, our ancestors and our blood. It is the energy that inhabits the trees and is responsible for everything that happens on Earth.

Iroko

Iroko, you are ancestry
Your being is filled with
Energy, wisdom and vitality
Powerful avatars
we got in the beginning
Full of talents and generous heart,
Sprouting from your rich branches
From the robust and mighty trunk,
With incredible latent power
The roots that hold
the secrets of humanity
The past,
the present
and the future
More than just a sublime sign
Of divine arboric essence
You are worthy of all
the praise and reverence
Gloriously empowering us
to love and to live

Sandra de Moura

BREATHING

The air element
The breath
The metaphor of the deities

We openly invite you to think with us and draw your own conclusions.

If you're alive, you're breathing.
The first thing you do after your born is breathe.
The last thing one does is to take their last breath.
Without air, the body dies and ceases to function, the 5 senses are void!

Breathing and breathing without obstruction, you are able to control parts of your involuntary bodily function. You are able to regulate control of your breathing and calm the bodies systems of physiological response. This is a basic principle of an stable equillibrium.

Breathing is an automatic function. To take control over the act of breathing can only be done for a limited time. It is possible to control breathing for some minutes, it is also possible to stop breathing for a while, but in the absence of breathing, if only for a few minutes, can cause irreparable brain and cellular lesions.

Knowing how to breathe and paying attention to our own breathing lets us experience health and tranquility. The mix of healthy breathing and calculated movements brings many benefits to the body and to the mind. For millennia, entire civilizations have practiced use of these principles.

Nothing happens on the face of our planet, without interaction with the air. We are immersed in this atmosphere. Other elements, such as fire, water and earth, can not manifest without it.

So here are some basic breathing exercises for any time you are feeling tensions, anxieties, or sadness.

If you are in a small or a big imbalance. If you are preparing for the exercises in this book or you are in a traffic jam or an accident.

If you are waiting for someone to arrive or for your turn in line.

If you are before a medical examination, or in the park about to ride the roller coaster.

Doesn't matter where, but always remember, **BREATHE**!

SOME BREATHING EXERCISES

CIRCLE BREATHING

Take a deep breath at 1, keep on breathing in until 4, pay attention to pause, exhale at 1, keep exhaling until 4, regular doing so until calm or anxiety goes away.

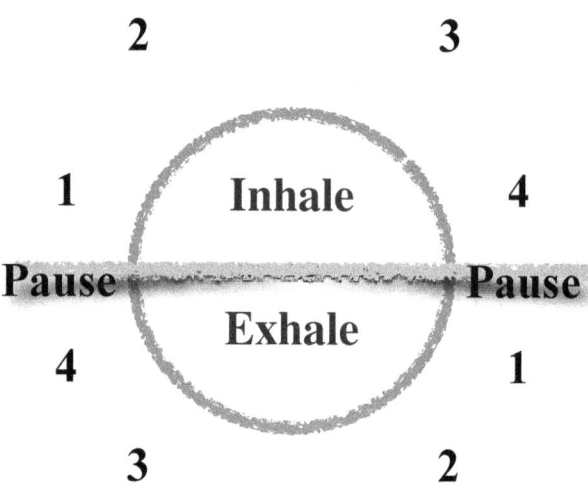

Heart Coherence

This is an exercise based on research of the *HeartMathInstitue.com*, where professionals, such as Doctors and Psychologists, study the theme and its effects of mental and physical health, and also in a description from the book, „Anti-Anxiety toolkit", from Melissa Tiers.

Put all your attention in your hearth. Imagine yourself breathing deeply, in and out of your chest.

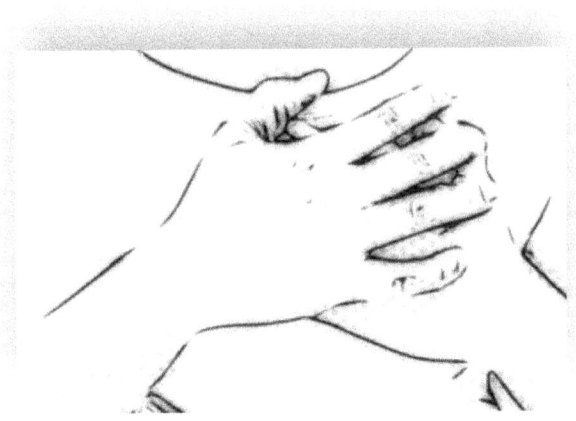

Hold your hand over your heart to keep your attention on it. As you keep on repeating, imagine your heart pumping the best quality blood in your whole body and radiating energy through your whole being.

After doing this exercises for a while, your brain waves will find theirselves in a better brain waves state.

Bi-Neural Breathing

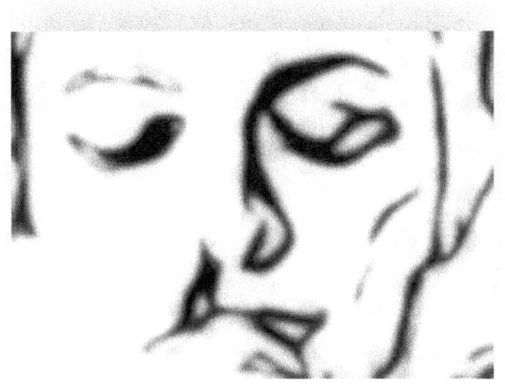

Rest your right ring finger and thumb on either side of your nostrils, lightly touching them but not constricting. Take a big breath and exhale, then close off the right nostril with your thumb and inhale through the left nostril fully for a count of four. At the climax of that breath, close off the left nostril with your ring finger, hold your breath for a count of four, and then release the right nostril and exhale for a count of four.

Next, inhale deeply for a count of four through the right nostril, close it off, hold your breath for a count of four, and then release the left nostril as you exhale completely through for a count of four.

Proceed to repeat the cycle.

Do this as many rounds as you like, being sure to exhale through the left nostril to complete your last cycle.

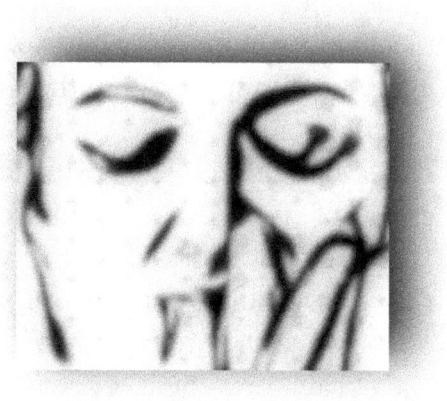

Wellbeing
Exercises

THE AWAKENING

Every cell, a world!
Every individual, the cosmos!
From this premise arises the responsibility for each act.
Self-improvement is proof of spiritual maturity.
To recognize this purpose is, at the same time, to release the reins of the control of tomorrow and to act in the now, is to know that we are particles of an All and that, when we ascend, we influence our environment.

THE ELEMENTS:

AIR, WATER, EARTH AND FIRE

Are significant tools that can help us manage the journey of life.

The effects they have on us can be enjoyed in a practical, fast and constant way. For the exercises, we reserve only a few minutes in our routine.

They can be performed in any order or energy imbalance. Feeling the vibrations of each element unites us with the Source of our existence .

Starting from these principle, we will use the properties of each element to enhance our homeostasis.

In conjunction with the breathe we will produce a synergetic experience.

AIR

Air, breath, life-force whatever one calls it, air is a constant presence in all aspects of life. Air element is part of all the elements and exercise. Air element can be considered the most important. Breath through the nostrils, mouth closed, fill the belly with breath, slow and deep. We focus equally on the inhale and exhale, depending on the energetic effect we want. We will make-longer exhalation, and or longer inhalations and it can become an act of meditation, physical mantra, or preparation for meditation.

IROKO TREE

Iroko tree is the source of our inspiration, grounded to earth, but continually reaching its branches up and out to the heavens. We use the Iroko tree as a metaphor for our lives.

The Iroko tree is the basis for all exercises, and has a connection to all elements: it cleanses our air, the water enlivens our bodies. The earth grounds us and gives nourishment, and fire is fuel for new beginnings.

All exercises should be started from the Iroko Tree stance.

Use full inhales and exhales to complete cycles of exercises, 5 reps.

On each side completes the exercise.

If bending knee, no knees over toes.

Please, take care of your body, don't over do it!

Please consult your Physician before starting any new exercise program.

Iroko (Tree of ancestors)

Starting alignment-Standing, feet hips distance apart, palms open facing forward at your sides, spine long, shoulders relaxed and pulled back, gaze straight ahead

Description of movement

Start inhale, heel toe feet outside of hips to a 45 degree angle, raise arms into a V-pattern fingers pointing towards right angle on ceiling, twisting edge of hands to the sky, exhale twisting edge of hand towards back wall and lowering chin.

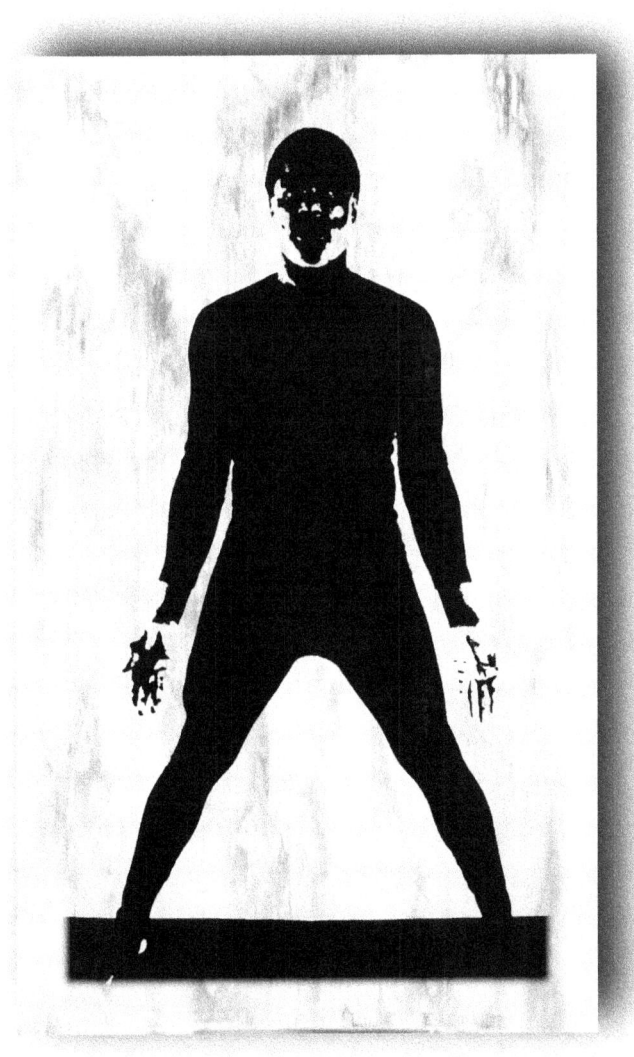

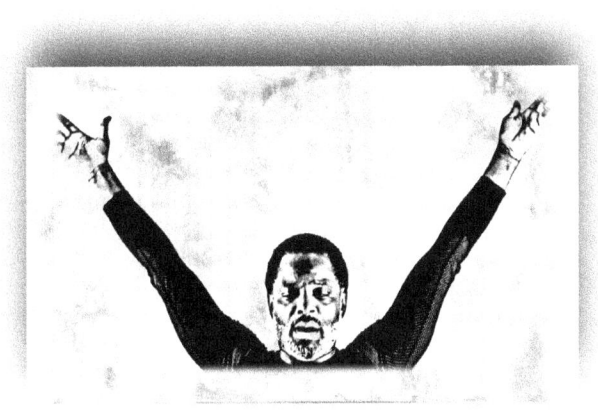

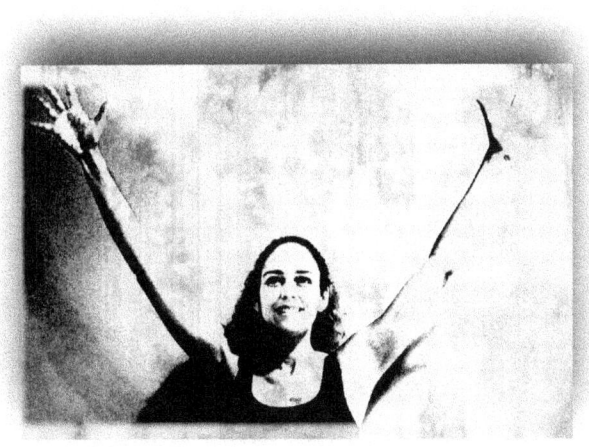

WATER

Water has many facets, oceans, seas, rivers, lakes, streams, and ponds.

Water also has varying temperament, and can be calm, placid, whirling, rushing, unpredictable.

However, it can gives us surprising effectiveness.

It's liquid nature helps us smooth out the rigidity in our physicall body, and makes our mind more pliable.

Its effectiveness can be measured by mind to body connection, a calm mind and a balanced body or a calm body and balanced mind.

Ocean tide

Starting alignment
Iroko tree position

Description of movement

Bring arms down to your sides, step your right foot to the right, the length of one of your legs, turning right foot at a 90 degrees.

Left foot facing forward, inhale while bending into right knee, keeping left leg straight, twisting hips to the right and raising arms to the sky. Slight backbend. Exhale slowly swing arms down while straightening and return right foot forward.

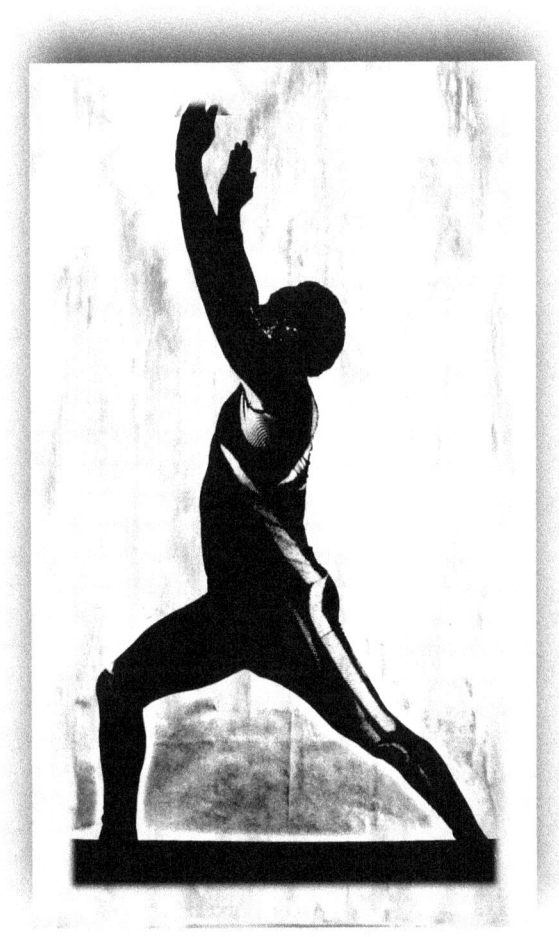

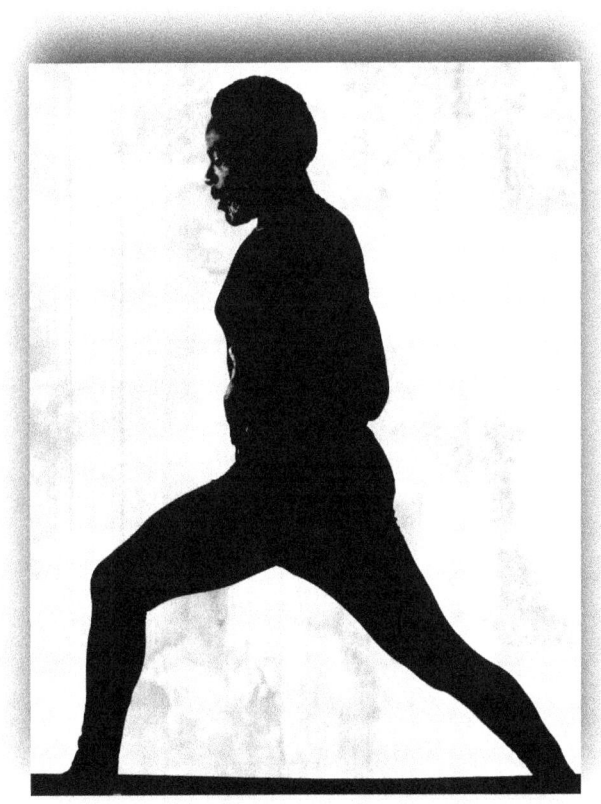

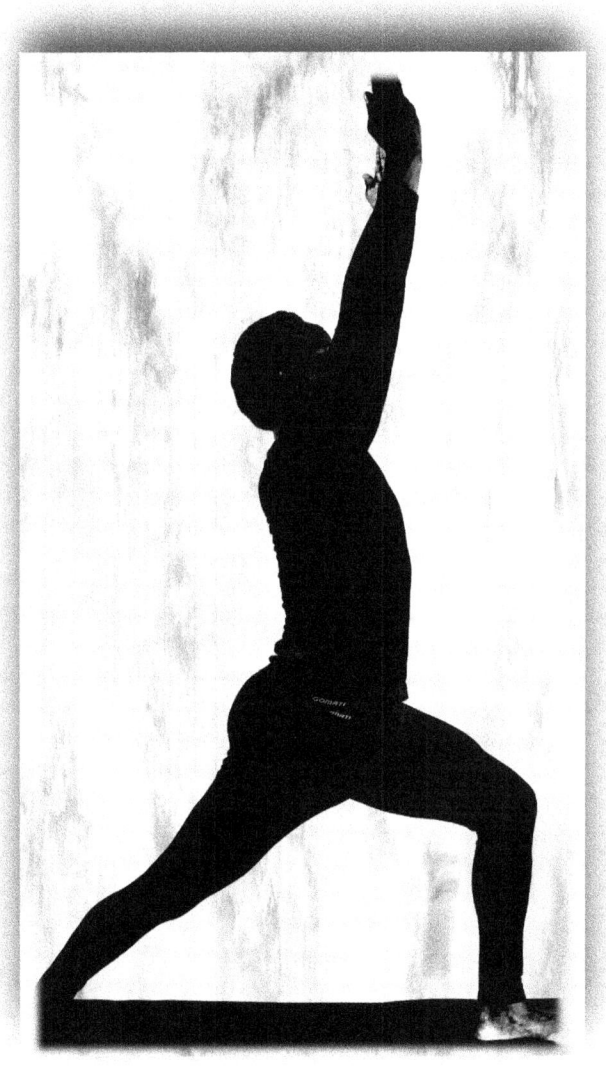

Upwelling
(Water II)

Starting alignment
Iroko tree position

Description of movement

Bring legs together, start to exhale, keep gaze forward, while bending to a squat, your arms come down in front of you.

Inhale, straightening legs and swinging arms out and up (if possible on tiptoe).

With the arms, we imitate breast swimming, moving arms in circles.

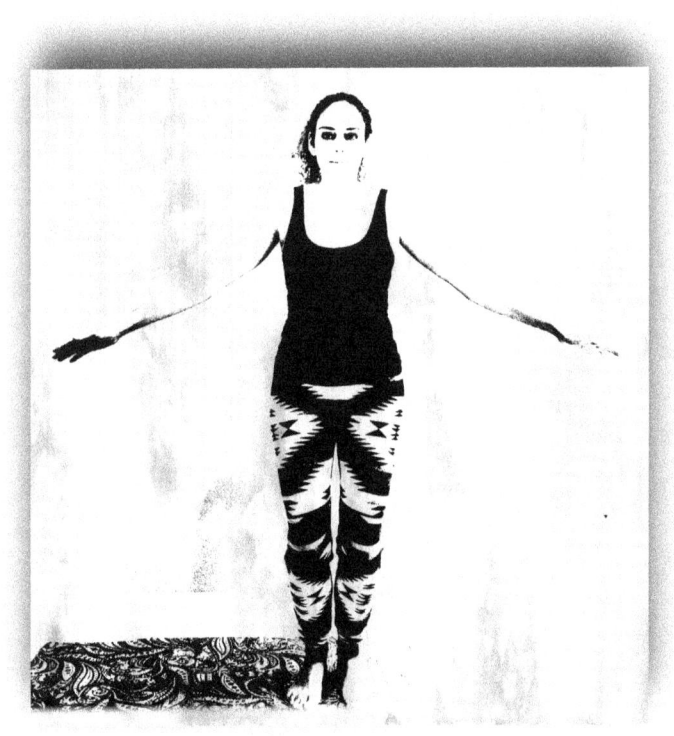

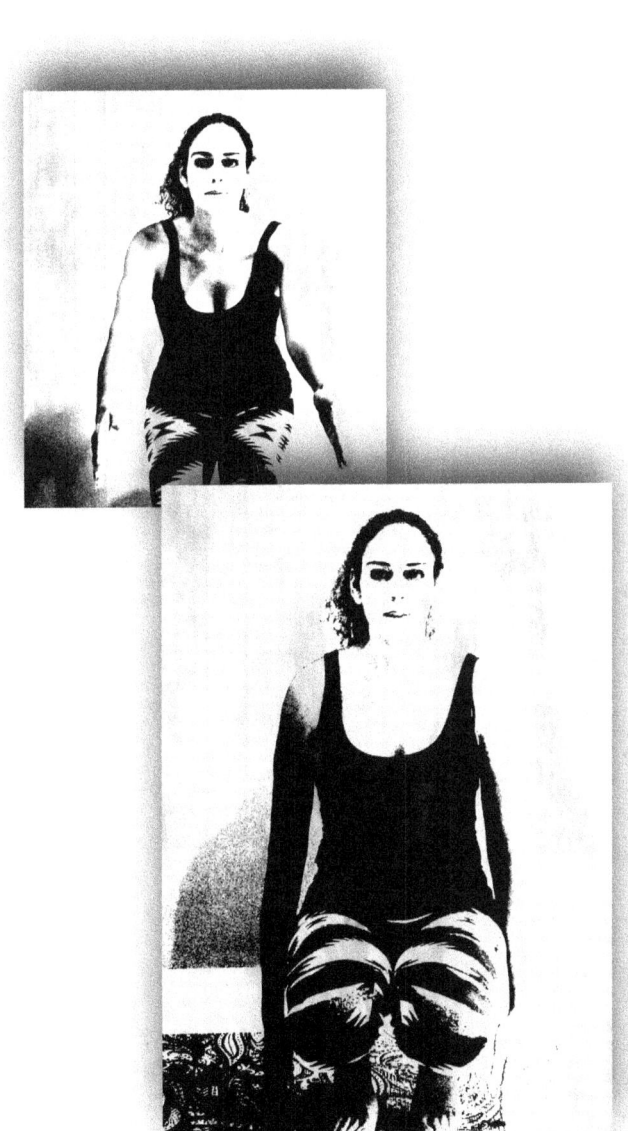

69

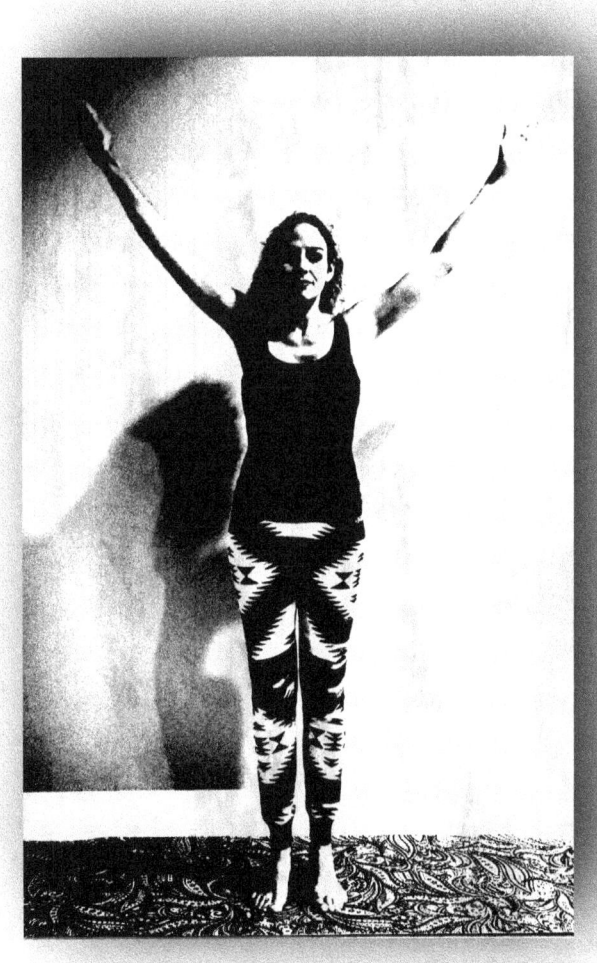

EARTH

Foundation and roots can be used to symbolize a solid place to build.

Earth confirms our humanity. Like roots underground we stabilize ourselves by connecting to earth and each other.

Earth exercises gives us stability.

Praying flower
(Earth 01)

Starting alignment
Iroko tree position

Description of movement

Come to sit with top of feet on floor and hands resting at your sides, palms up. Inhale, lifting hips forward, while stretching arms towards the sky, slight backbend.

Exhale, return hips back to starting point.

Pull belly to spine, fold forward, bringing arms down to the floor, palms open. Head and arms in alignment.

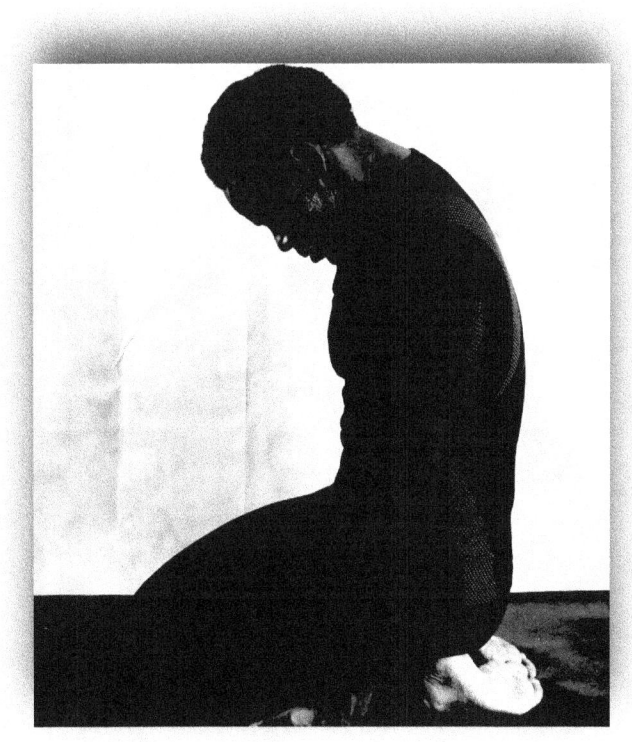

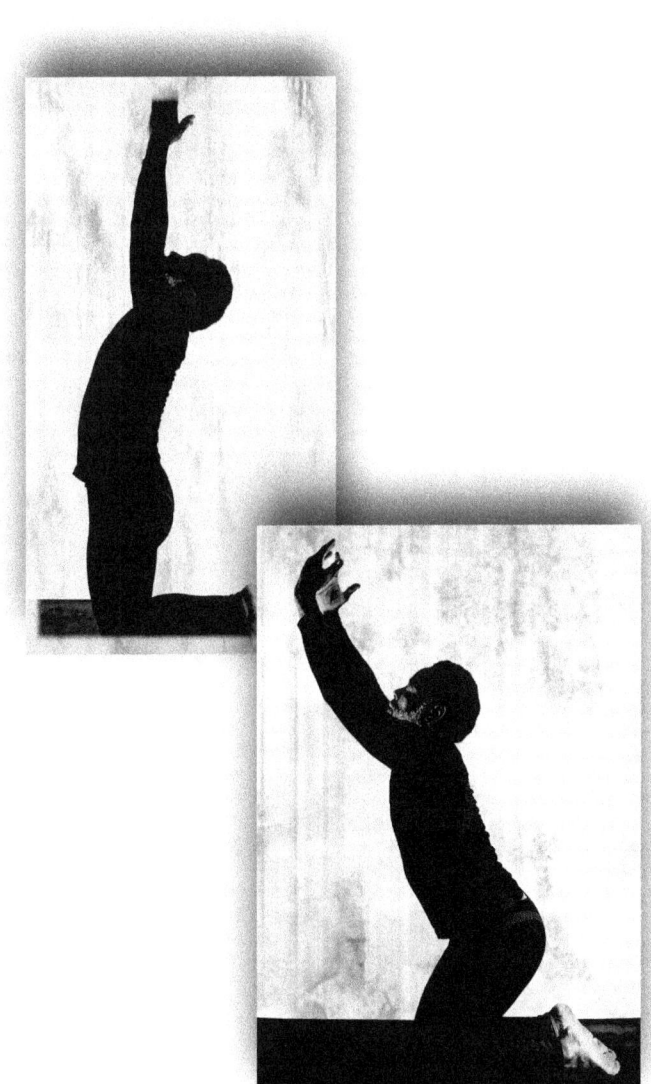

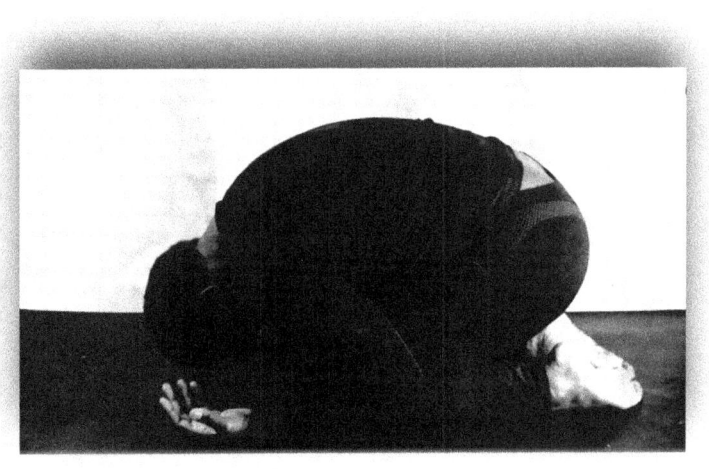

4 point clover

Starting alignment
Iroko tree position

Description of movement

We stand on tiptoes, bending knees outward, keeping torso upright and, with our knees far apart, we sit upon our heels.

Dropping our arms along our backside as we touch the ground with our outstretched fingers.

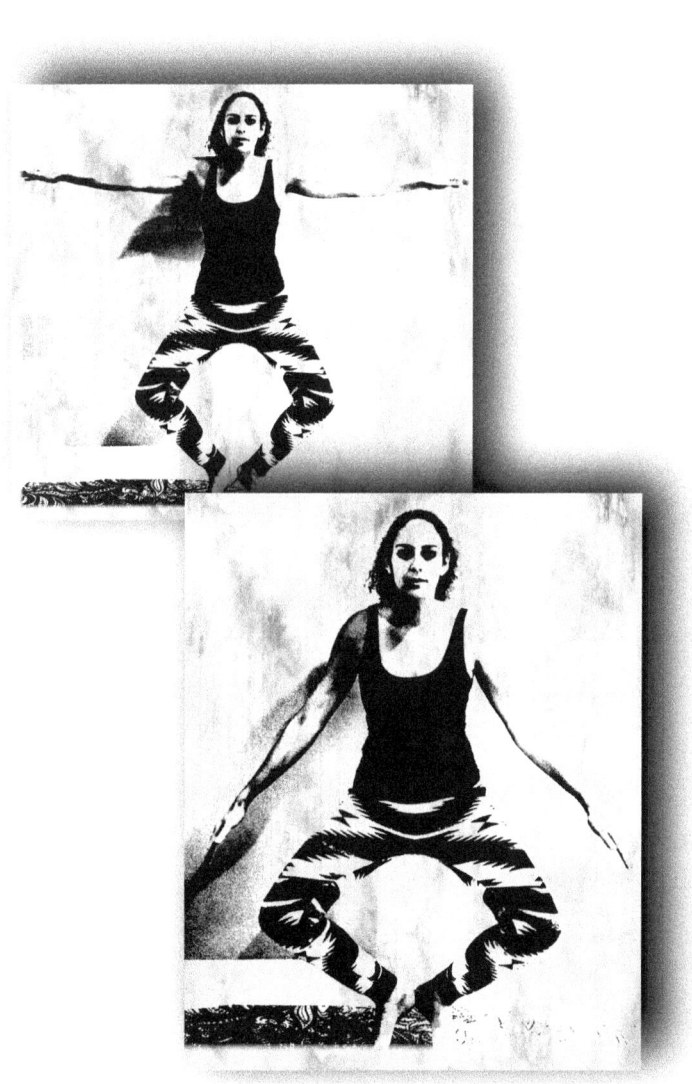

85

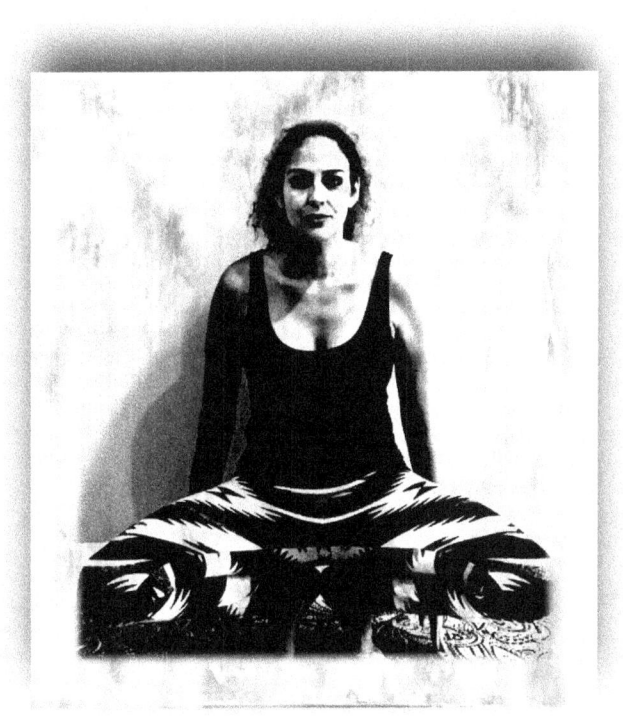

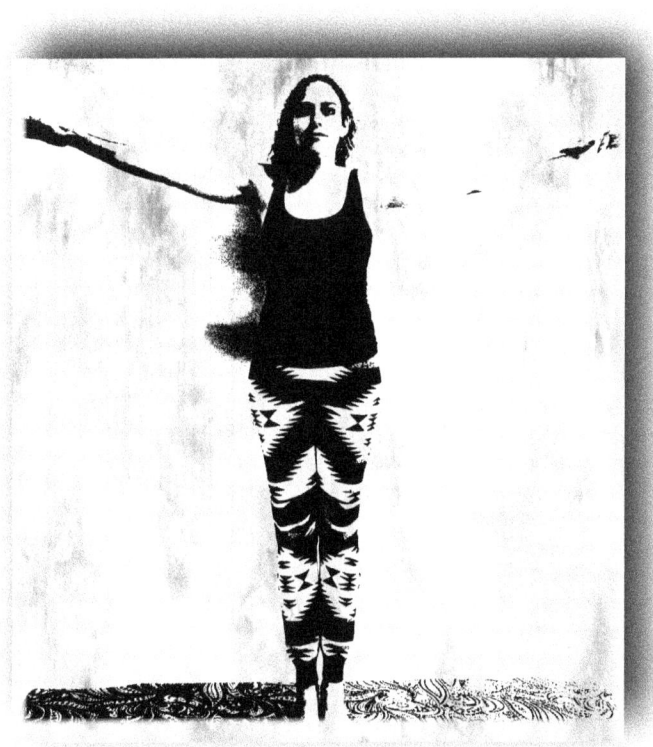

FIRE

Fire is the fuel to power our bodies and minds, stored in our core, supplied by the sun.

Energy to create new, and extinguish what does not serve us.

Fire motivates us against lethargy and manipulative influences. With great power comes great responsibility!

Be cautious!
This energy has no limits,
fuel the good in yourself.

Bellows

Starting alignment
Iroko tree position

Description of movement

Arms to your side knees sightly bent, Inhale, chest forward, tilt head back, push hips and butt backwards and up.

Exhale, push pelvic forward, pull belly to the spine, shrug shoulders forward, chin to chest.

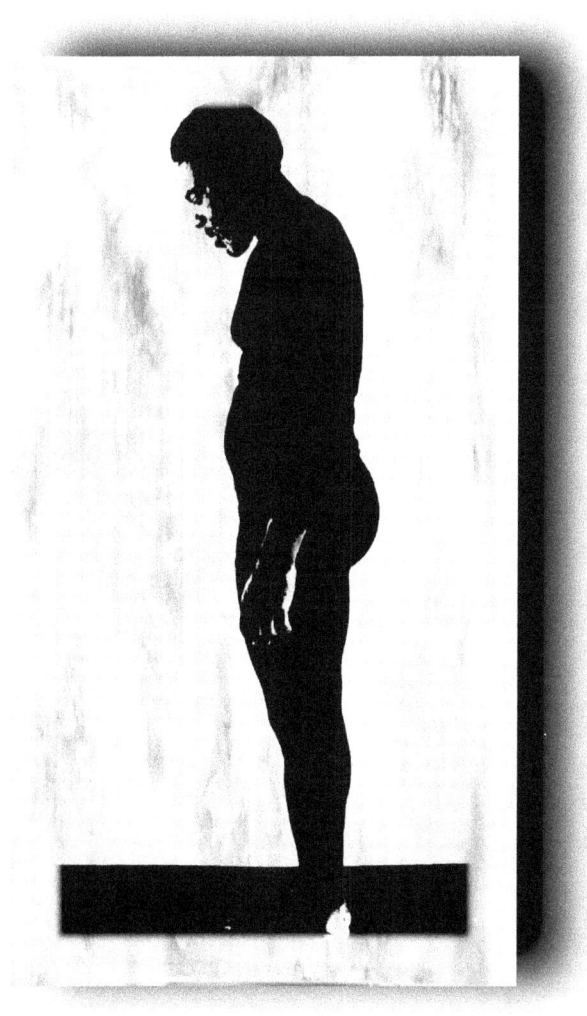

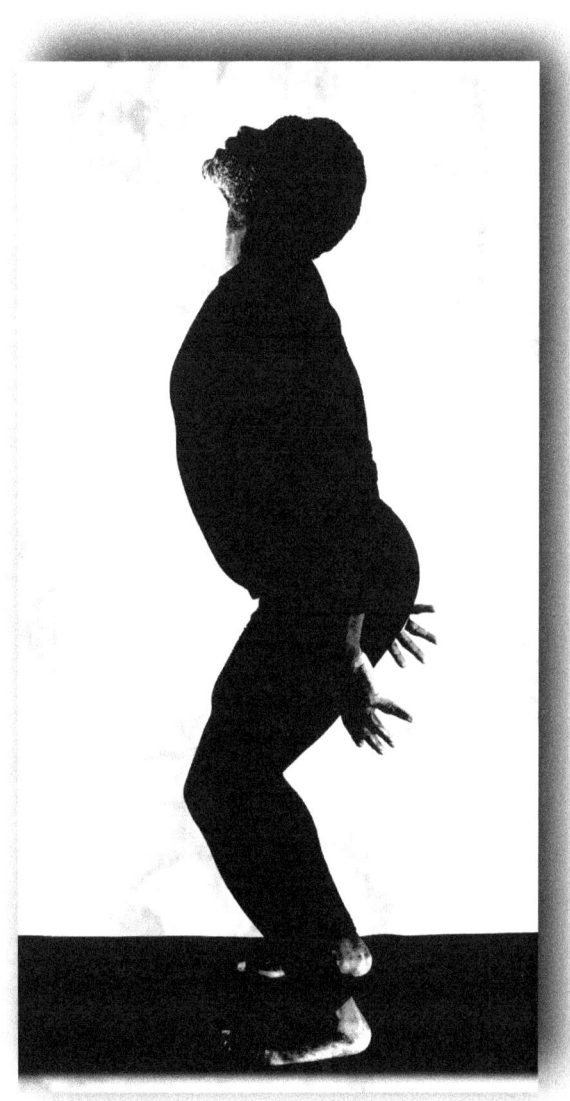

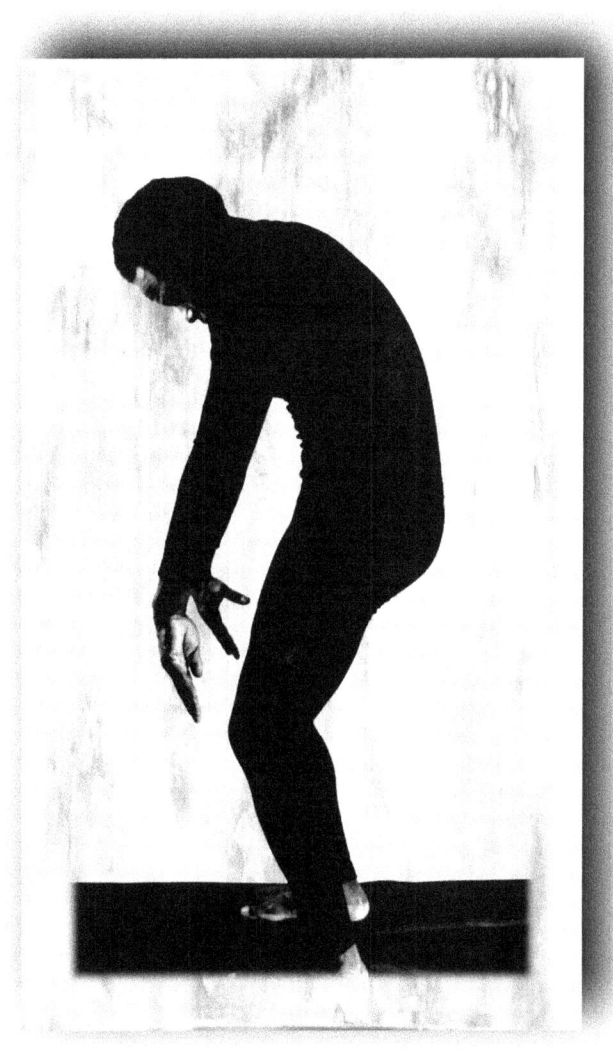

Flame

Starting alignment
Iroko tree position

Description of movement

Standing with our feet together, we start to inhale while we left our arms to the sky in a V-formation, lifting chest, slight backbend.

Exhale slowly, pulling belly button back to spine, while curling torso into a ball, wrap arms around back giving yourself a big hug, lower chin to chest.

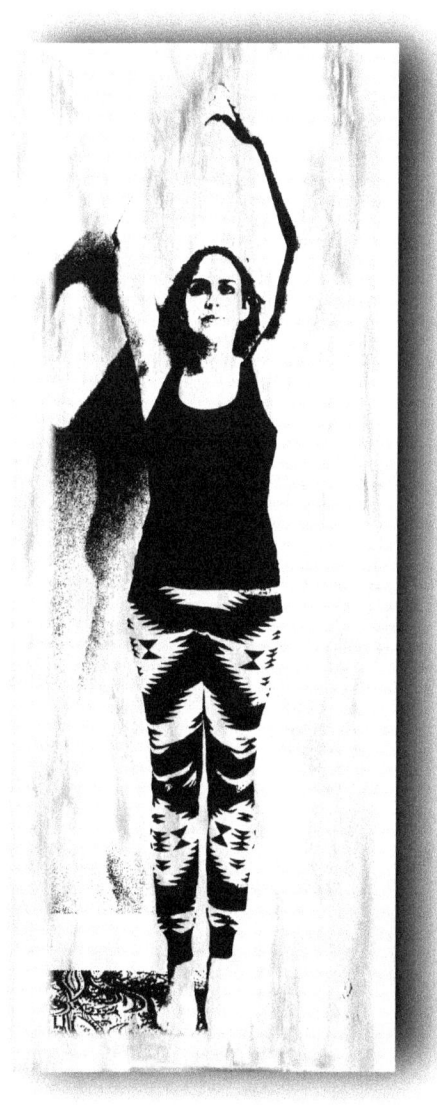

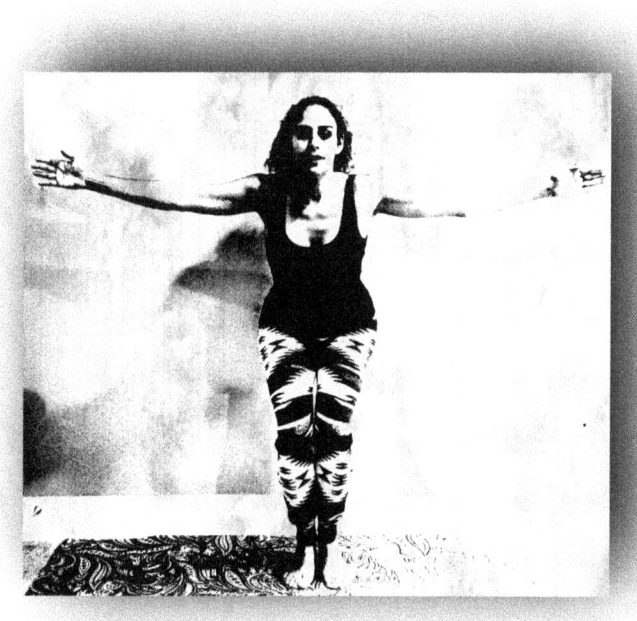

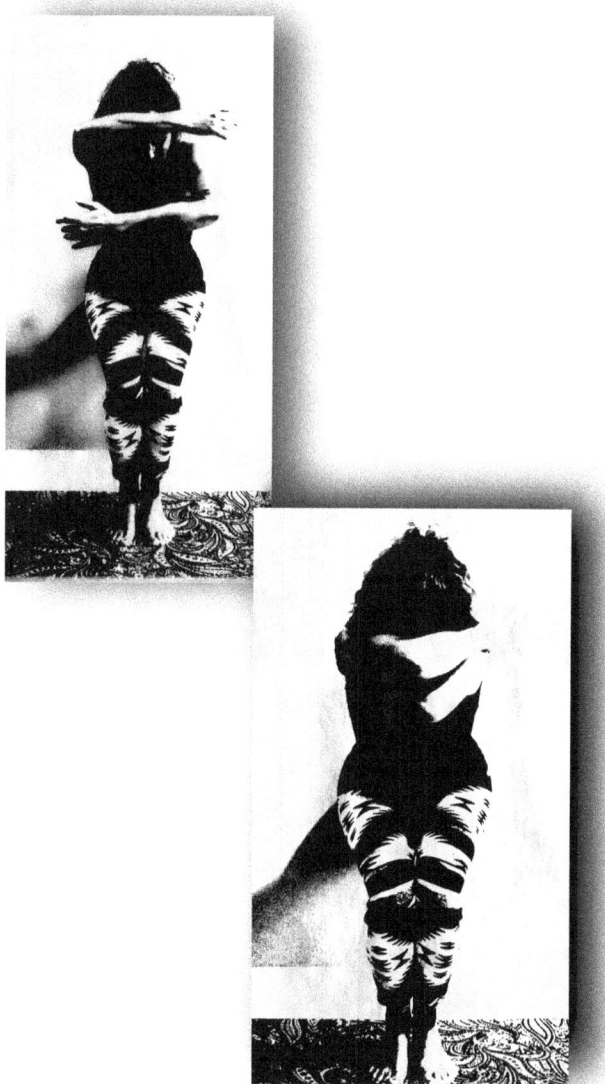

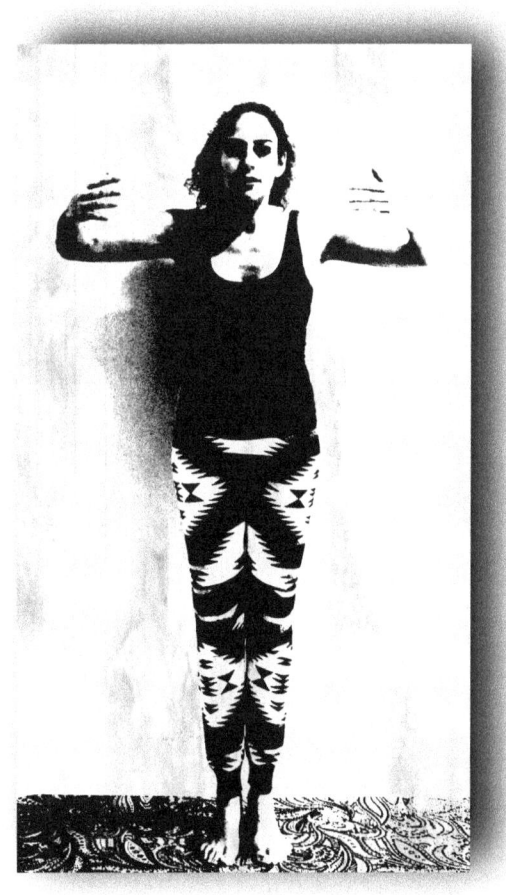

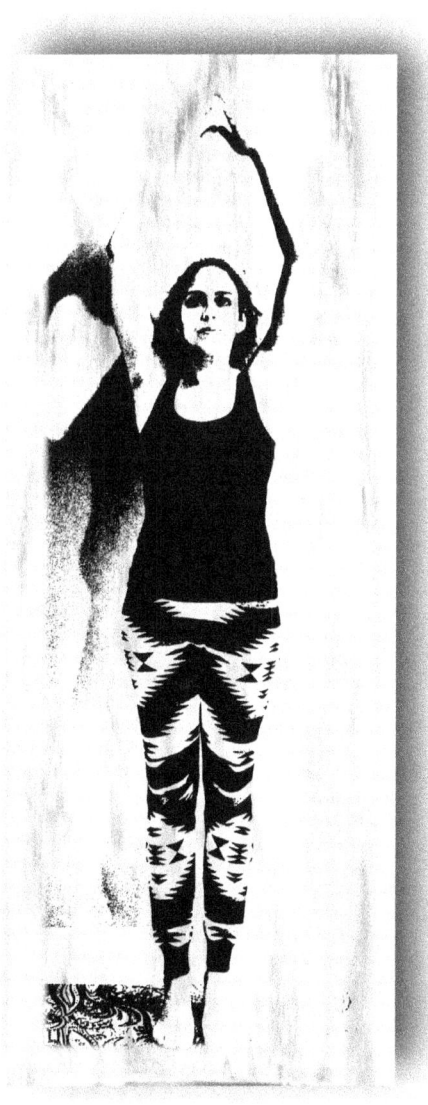

How to reach us:

Germany:
Postfach 600 129
70301 Stuttgart

USA

PO BOX 52035
Palo Alto, California
USA, 94303

Sandra De Moura:
omsandrademoura@gmail.com

Rondy Isaac:
balancemakerri@gmail.com

Ligia Braz:
Ligia@brasiversum.com

**Thank you so much
for your time
and support!**

We see you!

Peace, Health & Iroko!

Sandra

Ligia

Rondy

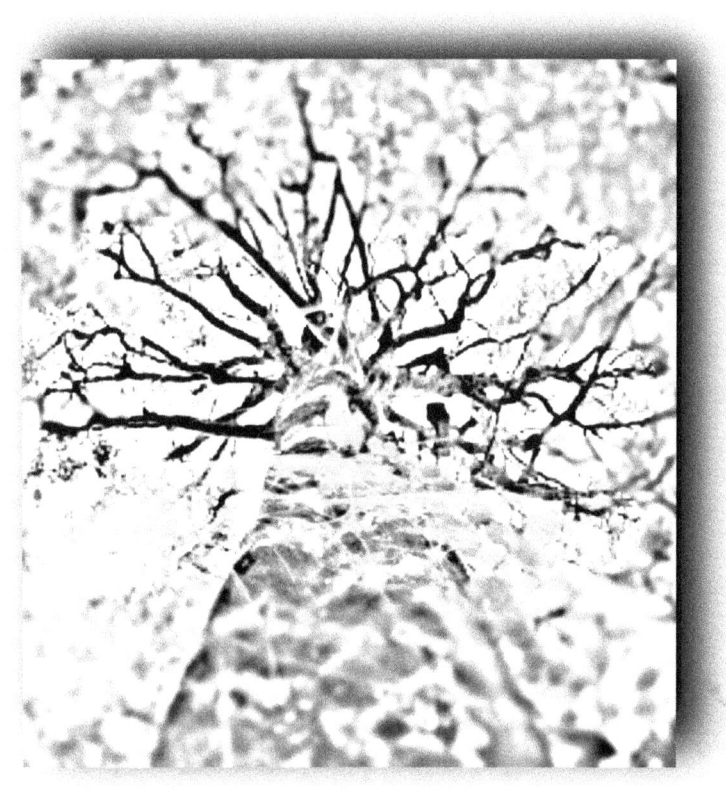

www.ingramcontent.com/pod-product-compliance
Lightning Source LLC
Chambersburg PA
CBHW060412290526
45791CB00002B/710